100 Ways
TO LIVE A

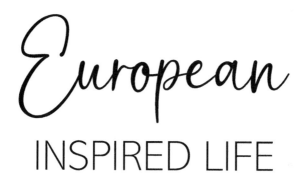

INSPIRED LIFE

FIONA FERRIS

Contents

100 Ways to Live a European Inspired Life 7

50 more ways to bring a little European flair into your life 74

About the Author 89

Other books by Fiona Ferris 91

FIONA FERRIS

Dear lovely reader,

I know, I know, the French Chic thing has been covered *a lot* over the past couple of decades. But you're here reading this and I'm here writing it so there must still be something in it for a lot of us. Words and ideas still to be shared. Inspiration to be had. If only for simple happiness and *joie de vivre* ('cheerful enjoyment of life'). What inspires us, inspires us.

The fact is, romantic souls like ourselves love the fanciful notion of *acting as if* we live in France, even Paris, and in doing so sprinkling a little French fairy dust over our everyday lives. Or perhaps we live in Tuscany in our mind. We don't care that it's not 'real', that actual Parisiennes would never do many of these things (or would they?) and may even chuckle at the thought of people in other countries pulling on a beret, or breaking a chunk of baguette off for lunch.

None of this matters to me. Firstly, if I were that

Parisienne, I'd be flattered if someone considered my lifestyle so enticing that they idealized it.

And for us, the dreamers and the doers, we get to live our life exactly as we want to – residing in the house that we do, with the people we love, going to our job, participating in social events and enjoying our downtime. But we get to do all of this with an added *frisson*, a little tingle of excitement as we elevate our daily activities by viewing them through a stylish Euro-tinted lens.

As much as I adore the essence of France, my heart is also taken by Italy. There is just something about Italian style that is more accessible, warmer, and down-to-earth too; sexier, less buttoned up. And when I think about my favourite foods, Italian cuisine is right up there. Italy is the secret sister for me, and she guides me in a way that I don't always appreciate.

I have only visited Italy once – Rome, for a mere two or three days – but it made a big impact on me and I can still remember the details. How confident and flamboyantly dressed the women were, and the sense of personal style so important to Romans. The smartly dressed young men and women zipping around on Vespas, coffee balanced on the handlebars and held precariously with one hand. The espresso bars everywhere.

And Paris, it was for a similar short amount of time, but I'm so glad I got to stroll around and soak in her beauty.

My main inspirations are Italian and French; you

may be the same or perhaps the Spanish way of life is what appeals to you most. South American cultures are similar too. No matter your flavour, this book will ignite your creativity to create *your* version of a European-inspired life.

It's so much fun having an active imagination don't you think? That you almost feel sorry for people who are more 'normal' in how they view things? Do you think they get as much enjoyment from everyday living as we do? I highly doubt it! It's like having a fun and inspiring movie running in your mind every day, and *it's wonderful.*

Don't let other people tell you how to live, to be more realistic, and to not be so frivolous. Don't let them rain on your parade. Instead, zip all your deliciousness up into your secret garden and enjoy living your best European-inspired life. No experience necessary.

We get to design a life that thrills us from every angle. Why would we deprive ourselves of that? It makes no sense. So if you're just as happily 'delusional' as me, follow along for a fun trip to fill your life with fanciful delights and French- and Italian-inspired happiness. We're going to have so much fun.

And I promise, you will be brilliantly inspired to add a little European flair into *your* everyday life by the end of this petite book. I know because I found it for myself as I wrote and edited it. By the final pages I was so pumped to be even more *euro chic* than I am already. And my health and lifestyle goals were effortlessly achieved too which was a nice surprise. I'm sure it will be the same for you.

Let's meet at that chic little café on the corner and I'll share all my ideas with you. I'll see you inside!

With all my best from a warm spring day in beautiful Hawke's Bay, New Zealand,

Fiona

100 Ways to Live a European Inspired Life

1. **Capture the details**. Start a list of all the little things you might like to include in your European-style life going forward. As you come across ideas write them down. It might be new ways to style your outfits gleaned from a fashion blog. Or when there is a French Chic flat-lay in a fashion magazine and you soak in every detail – make a note of the elements that stand out for you. Is it the colour palette? Specific accessories? Or maybe you will make a note of lifestyle habits you want to pick up such as eating dinner later and having an *aperitivo* (early evening drink) and chat before that. For me, I wanted to wear brighter colours, accessorize in gold jewellery, and live life more lightly. With your 'new' Euro-

inspired life *include every detail that makes your heart happy.* You owe it to yourself!

2. **Live the way you want to live**. Only you get to decide if you want to live a prettier life and have a more pleasurable daily experience. No-one else can give it to you; you must claim it. And since you're reading this book, it will likely be a French-inspired, European-style life that you covet. It's your happy place. But your happy place could just as easily be plant-based healthy living, craft-craft-craft, or super minimalist, and you can infuse them all together with your European fantasy existence. Claim all the flavours you love and create your bespoke lifestyle. Make it fun. Enjoy every moment by surrounding yourself with what you love, to create your own unique flavour – a flavour that delights *you*.

3. **Include green in your décor**. The stereotypical French lady is said to pick up a bunch of flowers from her neighbourhood florist with which to beautify her parquet-floored apartment, and sometimes I do this, but I actually prefer silk flowers and good-quality *faux* plants. This is something I realized about myself only in recent times. I love the look of house plants and flowers, but the admin weighs me down *so much* – the watering and trimming, soil- or water-

changing, and vase washing. I found myself *not* having plants and flowers in the house because of these factors. Then I discovered high-quality alternatives. They might not be for everyone, but *I love them*. Find a nature touch that works for you – perhaps you love arranging flowers and tending to your potted plants and would never consider pretend options – and place one or two in each room.

4.   **Show the best version of yourself**. Italians call this concept *la bella figura*, which literally translates to 'the beautiful figure', but more often means *to put your best foot forward in everything you do*. I love this, because it means the aesthetic of every aspect of your life is considered: how you dress, how you live at home, how tidy and clean your car is... You want to make a good impression, and it all comes down to how you present yourself. Whether you are somewhere casual or more formal, you will be dressed appropriate to the occasion, and with a little flair too. When you present yourself well, you show that you have self-respect. That you hold yourself with pride and dignity. Borrow *la bella figura* from the Italian culture and elevate every category of your life with ease and pleasure.

5.   **Care for your skin**. Young girls in Europe are taught how to best look after their skin by

their mothers. I was lucky enough to have the same experience and it has served me well. It's as much as a habit as brushing my teeth twice a day. Whether you had a good start or not, *today* is the perfect time to upgrade your skincare regime (and by upgrade, I mean do it regularly, not rush out and buy pricey lotions – I prefer to use inexpensive drugstore products). And the best way to make it something you *want* to do, is to look at skincare as part of your pampering, luxurious, spa-like lifestyle. Washing your face at night, applying lotion all over after your shower, exfoliating and putting a mask on once a week; they are all forms of pleasurable self-care. And, when you give yourself the time to do it, will leave you feeling relaxed, calm, as well as giving you an outcome of having the best complexion you can as you get older.

6. **Set a beautiful table**. Create a delightful backdrop for your meal, whether it be breakfast, lunch, dinner, or even afternoon tea. Make it as simple or as fancy as you like. At a minimum I use a placemat, cloth napkin, porcelain dishes, and real cutlery. I have a small selection of dinner napkins that I have collected over the years, and I use them regularly. They get thrown in the wash with my tea towels and dish cloth. I also have a few dinner sets, and it's enjoyable to set a different

looking table than normal, especially when entertaining. Even if it's just for you, put out a placemat, choose a pretty plate, and set a glass of water down. Dine with *panache* and think of your *dolce vita* ('sweet life') as you close your eyes for a second before you eat.

7. **Try a European wine**. I mostly choose to purchase New Zealand wine to support the local economy, for the carbon footprint, and value too since it hasn't had to travel as far, but there is something quite thrilling about sipping a glass of French Rosé or Spanish Rioja. I think of everything those grapes went through to get to my glass, including a long boat trip. And thankfully, wine from Europe is available at all price points, even everyday quaffing prices. To elevate your experience even more, watch documentaries or vineyard tours set in France or Italy. I find it fascinating that 'old world' European wines are named for the area in which they are grown, such as Bordeaux, Chablis, or Champagne, whereas 'new world' wines from North America, Australia, and New Zealand, for example, are named for the grape varietal: Sauvignon Blanc, Shiraz or Chardonnay, etc. And pouring a glass of Ultimate Provence Rosé, which, while more than my usual wine budget, is special to sip and I can appreciate where it came from. It is a little taste of Provence for far

less than the cost of a plane ticket (and the bottle is beautiful enough to use again afterwards).

8. **Elevate your non-alcohol game**. If you are not a drinker, pick up a bottle of Lemon Perrier sparkling water, or Sanpellegrino Aranciata Rossa (blood orange). I mostly drink New Zealand sparkling water for the same reasons as choosing New Zealand wine, but when we have a bottle of plain Sanpellegrino on the table like last night it feels different. (I decided that Saturday night was worthy of a 'treat' bottle of sparkling water.) These European drinks are more expensive than local options, but I justify them to myself that they are still a lot cheaper than purchasing alcohol, and I don't have them every night.

9. **Curate your makeup collection**. No matter how much or how little makeup you use, you will likely have more than you need. My makeup selection has been downsized over the years and I love to use things up, but there is always further to go I have found. Just last week I threw out two eyeshadow palettes. They were both inexpensive. One was a well-used favourite but the lid was cracked and fell off all the time, and the other was a disappointment in that the pigments were so faint that they needed heavy application to show. And in the

meantime, I wasn't using a more expensive makeup set that I'd bought three years ago. Just what special occasion was I saving it for? The expired makeup party? So I threw out those two and now use my high-quality palette every day because I have no other option. It feels good not only to get use from the fancy palette, but also to have streamlined my makeup for an easier morning routine.

10. **Dress well at home**. It is important to be a well-dressed woman at all times, not just when you are going out. When I have a day of writing and home tasks and no plans to go beyond the gate, I still dress in a comfortable, clean, stylish outfit, do my hair, and put on a little makeup. It just feels better. And once it became a habit it didn't take any more time either. In fact, I'd say that doing this *saves* time, because when you look good and are well put together you feel more productive. You move with brisk purpose as well as feeling relaxed and happy while you do your chores. And, if someone knocks on the door, you are happy to open it. The trick is to dress as early in the morning as possible so you can enjoy the benefits all day. Can you imagine your dream Parisian self slouching around in leggings and a sweatshirt with messy hair and no makeup? No, she is dressed and active, making the most of her day, and looking cute while she is at it.

11. **Go to film festivals when they are on**. As I write this, I have a program for the *Cinema Italiano Festival* on my desk. It's exciting to peruse through and see what films look appealing, and it also brings back happy memories of foreign films I have been to in the past. It feels so good to leave a theatre after a particularly affecting movie, and you can't help but be uplifted after a joyous viewing. And the bad ones, well, they're best forgotten about but even then, you get to see another point of view. If you don't have anything foreign coming to your local theatre, see what's available on your streaming services and dip into another culture, with subtitles of course.

12. **Commit to one thing**. There will likely be areas in your life that could be better; make a list of everything you'd love to improve. Then choose one or two that will make *the most* difference to your enjoyment of life and commit there and then to make an everlasting change that will take you where you want to go. It might be your weight, taking care of your money, organizing your home, or enhancing a relationship. *You are the one driving the bus.* If there is something you truly dislike, focus on making small actions every day to improve your situation. Keep your attention on the daily habits, not some far-off outcome. And never give up. Prove to yourself that you have

the ability to change. What I admire about the European people I know personally, is that they are very matter of fact. If there is something they don't like, they change it, and without drama too. They don't seem to feel stuck. They just do it. So simple!

13. **Choose experiences over things**. For the most part, Europeans have smaller homes and less possessions than those in other cultures. They don't feel the need to fill their space with more; instead they go out for a coffee, to dinner, a movie, an exhibition at an art gallery, or for a stroll around the park or city. Consider a 'consumable' outing over an 'accumulating' outing, unless you really do need to purchase a specific item of course. Often shopping is just a fun habit, but that's how we end up with a home filled with items we don't even use, and clutter that stresses us out. I often make it a goal to return home from a trip into town empty-handed. I know that sounds crazy, but it's enjoyable to see how much fun I can have while spending the least. It's not only satisfying, but I don't have to look for a space for my new doodad either.

14. **Tidy and simplify your home**. Look at radically reducing the inventory your home holds. Be inspired by homes in magazines and on Pinterest. I know they're staged homes, and

these homes are *always* perfect, but the images can reignite your desire to live in a more intentional way. Having fewer possessions epitomises the European way of life to me. European homes are often quite small, and there is no room for excess stuff. But what replaces 'the stuff' is an easier, calmer lifestyle, more time to read, relax and *just be*, and the time and energy to get together with friends. The less time you need to spend organizing your home, the more time there is to *live well*.

15. **Adopt olive oil as your beauty secret**. I once read that Sophia Loren used olive oil to moisturize her skin. Whether this is true or not it has always stuck with me and so olive oil has taken on a glamorous allure in my mind and I have made it my own personal beauty secret. I put a tablespoon in my morning smoothie. I use it as a facial cleanser, massaged in and removed with a hot, wrung-out face flannel. I toss steamed vegetables in a splash of olive oil and they taste delicious. I use it as a cuticle oil, apply it to my shins for a healthy sheen in the summer, and as a facial mask or even as a night-time moisturizer. I'm sure this is just a tiny portion of beauty treatments that olive oil can be used for. You will find many more if you search online. And, each time you use olive oil to enhance your health and beauty, picture

yourself as a modern-day Sophia Loren!

16. **Dedicate time to self-maintenance**. Picture the European you, regularly tending to her physical body with self-love and pleasure. Shaping and painting her nails once a week. Applying a face mask every Sunday morning. Shaving her legs and using self-tanner. Exfoliating in the shower and massaging in lotion afterwards. Putting sunblock on her décolletage to protect the delicate skin there from the sun. Booking in for a pedicure when she needs one, or doing it herself. Come up with an ideal schedule for yourself and see if you can make it happen. I have left my nails unpainted the last few weeks even though I normally like them polished. I had a lot of moving and packing to do to help a friend, but this is all finished now, so guess what I am looking forward to doing this afternoon?

17. **Be a savvy and chic fashionista**. Dressing well is so much more important in countries such as France and Italy. I observe it with people I know, and from social media. From what I have seen they buy designer goods more readily and spend money on high-quality clothes. I prefer to be a little more... thrifty, so I like to purchase mostly inexpensive or moderately priced clothing and adorn my outfit with one or two designer accessories. If I

am wearing a pair of well-fitting skinny jeans and a pretty top with my Chanel sunglasses, do you think anyone is going to notice that my clothes cost less than $100 for both pieces?

18. **Never be in a hurry**. Even if it means you might be a few minutes late, stop to give someone the time of day. Simplify your schedule so you can feel relaxed and at ease and not have to rush from one appointment to the next. You may change nothing else but your mindset too, from one of 'go, go, go' to 'I have an abundance of time'. I often find that when I rush, I forget to take things with me, I make more of a mess, or I break something. It may well be one of life's paradoxes that when we go slower we can go faster. Europeans already know this. They move at a slower pace than we do while focusing on what is most important, and enjoy life more as a result.

19. **Lean towards the Mediterranean diet**. Dine elegantly and feel healthier at the same time by focusing on fruits and vegetables, fresh fish, olive oil, yoghurt, and raw nuts. This way of eating draws from countries surrounding the Mediterranean Sea, such as France, Italy, Spain and Greece and is said to promote good health and a long life. Plus, it is delicious and looks *très stylish*. It really ticks all the boxes for those of us who desire to be a little more

European in our daily life. Serve chunky green olives as a snack, arrange sliced apple around a cheese platter, and pour yourself a small glass of red wine. Red meat and sweets are taken sparingly, and family mealtimes and daily activity are encouraged. As you can imagine, processed and snack foods are not in evidence with the Mediterranean diet (which I consider more a way to live rather than a 'diet' as we know the word). But would you want to anyway? There is nothing chic about processed food, or snacks straight from a rustly bag!

20. **Serve bread with a meal**. These days many of us are doing the low-carb thing, if not all the time it's at least on our minds, and bread often misses out. But there is something so rustic and appealing about fresh bread, olive oil to dip it into, and perhaps some dukkah too. When I travelled to Europe bread was served automatically at the everyday-style restaurants I dined at. In a restaurant recently I was presented with a small ramekin of beautiful quality olive oil, and it had a soft schmear of butter on the rim of the dish. With my butter knife I could serve a little of each onto my bread and it was such a nice touch. I have since decided there is nothing wrong with serving yourself a small piece of bread to enjoy with your meal (mine has to be gluten free sadly but it is still delicious to lightly toast one

slice and cut it into two triangles).

21. **Dream up your inner Italian girl** and do what *she* does to *bring her alive*. Here is mine for your inspiration, created from people I saw while in Rome, and notes from books and movies I have enjoyed. I write down all the little details and let them flavour my imagination. My inner Italian girl lives *la dolce vita* – 'the sweet life' and follows the *la bella figura* philosophy – making a good impression and putting her best foot forward in everything she does. In my mind she wears capri pants and a fitted blouse with ballet flats or tab-front loafers. Her wardrobe is minimal and stylish. She accessorizes with big sunglasses in black or tortoiseshell and carries a tote bag to pick up vegetables from the market. She dresses to show off her figure and to be seen. Chic sensual is her vibe. She strolls with her beau after dinner and says *buona sera* – 'good evening' to others. She sips espresso coffee or red wine at a charming side-street cafe or *ristorante*. She plays opera in her apartment while doing her housework. She is unabashedly feminine with a womanly figure and has big hair – straightened, and back-combed in a 1960s style. She rides a Vespa with her coffee balanced on the handlebars, wearing a pencil skirt, high heels, and an open-faced helmet. (I actually saw girls like this in Rome, it was a

treat for the eyes.) Of course, I'm not about to start backcombing my hair or even buying a Vespa, but it is certainly fun to have my Italian girl as a muse. She encourages me to loosen up, be peppier, and care less about what other people think of me. What about *your* muse? What does she like? Where does she live? How does she dress? What does she eat and drink?

22. **Generate your own family traditions**. Movie nights, make your own pizza, a walk after dinner, birthday meals, group vacations, Saturday afternoon coffee; there are so many ways you can enjoy family time and create beautiful memories for the future. Some of my favourite fun memories have been family occasions. Just being together is the best thing, and even if there might be a scrap every now and then, it's all part of being related to each other. It is fun to josh around, tease people good-naturedly, and have a laugh. Family time and family traditions are the most wonderful glue to hold you all together. And if your friends are your family, how lucky are you! All these traditions work equally well with dear friends!

23. **Master the art of happy hour**. Nothing says 'a life well lived' like sitting down for an hour or so before dinner with a cocktail and a bowl of olives. Or a glass of wine and a small

piece of cheese. In Italy it is called *aperitivo*, and in France, an *aperitif*. It is that time after work and before dinner to have a drink and catch up on your day with your friends or family. Choose a not-too-sweet drink (or sparkling water if you prefer) and let it whet your appetite for dinner while you bond and chat. Maybe you'll do this at home, or maybe you will partake in a bar. Wherever your happy hour happens to be, make sure to participate often. And if you are alone at this time, enjoy it with a book or magazine. Salut!

24. **Prioritize your lingerie drawer**. French ladies place a high emphasis on their lingerie, and I am all for this, but I come from a slightly more practical, thrifty angle. I am not going to buy a super-expensive bra and matching underwear, but I do like my bra and knickers to either match or complement each other. I make sure I am happy with my lingerie by going through it a few times a year too. Anything worn-out gets tossed, as do panties I just don't find comfortable. Life is too short! I buy a few new bras and top up my knickers at the same time. I go through different phases with my underwear. For a while I chose brightly coloured, lacy, sexy styles, whereas at the moment I am going for pretty, soft colours in comfortable knits. I like the 'invisible' seamless knickers that feel like you're wearing

nothing. This is just my current approach; work out for yourself your preferences and make sure you visit your underwear drawer regularly to ensure that you still enjoy wearing everything you have in there.

25. **Drink from beautiful glassware**. You wouldn't think that the glass you choose to sip from would make such a difference, but it does. Over the years I have inexpensively collected vintage stemmed water goblets from thrift stores to use for non-alcoholic drinks such as sparkling water or tonic. I am not precious about any of them, and they must be able to go through the dishwasher to earn a place on my shelf. I use *all* my glasses, from the cheapest to the most expensive. Otherwise, what is the point in having them? Yes, some have been broken, but that's the price you pay for living. Choose a 'special glass' tonight and you will see the subtle impact it makes on the enjoyment of your drink.

26. **Read novels set in Europe**. Transport yourself on an armchair holiday by reading a book set in your favourite European country. One such title for me was *When in Rome*, by Nicky Pellegrino. It is a fascinating and enjoyable read woven through the true story of the great tenor Mario Lanza when he and his family moved to Rome from the United States

to shoot a movie. The main character Serafina becomes his wife's assistant, so she has a behind-the-scenes view to this famous man. I remember almost sighing from happiness while reading; it felt like I was living right there in Rome with them, and I wanted to make more Italian dishes for dinner as a result. Ah bella, I was so sad to have finished, it was like the perfect evening out; you know there will be others, but this one was just so… divine. Sometimes a book finds you at exactly the right time and infuses its way into your very being. *Find those books for you* and indulge, often.

27. **Work on your outside and your inside simultaneously**. I love pairing personal development with personal style, and how it applies to creating a European-inspired life is simple. You upgrade your outfit choices and grooming standards to reflect the 'French you' or the 'Italian you', and at the same time you adopt an elevated mindset. You ask yourself: *What does she prioritize? Where are her boundaries? How does she hold herself?* When you polish the outside and the inside together is how you get ahead quickly and make quantum leaps in your advancement and happiness. Level up both at the same time to remain balanced and grounded. It's no use dressing in your nicer clothes if you carry the same 'woe is me' head around. And no-one will

get to see your brilliance if you create your new elevated mindset but take no time to put yourself together. You will find that when you dress better, you feel happier, so it helps when you want to improve your mindset. And vice versa. It's a perfect symbiotic arrangement to do both inner and outer upgrades together.

28. **Find your chic mentors**. I have a big list saved where I jot down my chic mentors and why I admire them. The attributes I attach to each person (whether I know them in real life, or they are famous people) show me where I desire to head towards. For example, I have Giorgio Armani as a mentor for his simplicity of line, unstructured way of dressing, simple and neutral colour palette, and fine Italian style. And Coco Chanel who was uniquely herself in a time of fussy dresses and hats and had a flair for designing and tailoring garments. She invented many iconic looks such as the Little Black Dress, produced stylish clothing from knit fabrics formally only used for underwear, and borrowed the masculine tweed jacket for ladieswear. People that you admire, write down little points about why you are drawn to them and enjoy cultivating those traits for yourself.

29. **Make the *passeggiata* a part of your life**. In southern parts of Italy there is a tradition

called 'passeggiata'; a leisurely evening stroll in the central plaza of town, where residents dress to see and be seen and socialize lightly with others. Doesn't this sound delightful? I like to take my *passeggiata* on a weekend, often Sundays, when my husband and I dress nicely but casually, and take the dogs for a walk along the waterfront, or window-shop in the art-deco city of Napier where we live. It's different to an exercise walk, it's more of a tourist amble where you enjoy your own town, get some fresh air, and maybe bump into people you know, or at the very least say 'Hello' to passers-by. Think what kind of *passeggiata* would fit best into your lifestyle and start to include it at least once a week. I think you will come to appreciate your new tradition too.

30. **Curate your Euro-style wardrobe**. Consider what you might wear in your idealized dreamy European life. Create a Pinterest board or write down your ideas and start bringing these details into your everyday life. For me, she would wear black, denim, simple lines, and classic pieces with a twist. She would have amazing hair – always clean and silky. People would know her for her gorgeous hair! She would keep to a simple makeup style and have a creamy complexion with matte red lipstick and lightly made-up eyes. Elegant gold jewellery would

complement her beauty. She would enjoy wearing bright colours in the summer and muted plums, camels and black in the winter. Whatever makes you feel chic and stylish, include that in your inspiration. A friend whose mother died a few years ago told me a wonderful piece of advice she had given her. 'As a woman gets older, dear, she should dress more like a French woman'. My friend said she was reminded of her mother's words when she saw I was wearing a blazer over my ripped jeans, with red shoes. I was quite tickled by that and thought it was a great piece of advice!

31. **Consider how the European you would differ**. It's quite a fun thing to consider. I asked myself how I would be subtly different if I lived in Italy; the idealized me of course, since I live in New Zealand. When you do this, you get all sorts of delicious inspiration to make your everyday life more fun and enjoyable. Here is mine: *I wear glamorous eye makeup. I make no apologies for my curves. I dress with a little bit of flamboyance and sexiness. I flirt in a playful and natural way, with both men and women. I look after my figure. I love being adventurous with new fruits and vegetables. I take time out to live my slow-paced European lifestyle. I care for my possessions. I savour a cup of coffee. I listen to opera. I have an exquisite complexion*

from using traditional products such as almond oil to cleanse my skin. I am sensual. Brainstorm a list of your idealized European self and start to live as her today. Enhance your already beautiful life with elements of the European you.

32. **Be a lady of feminine charm**. I could use a reminder of this just about *every other day*, since I am someone who often takes life too seriously and forgets how fun things can be when I lighten up. Life just gets so much better when you let yourself be sunny, flirty, and playful. When you don't stomp around being 'busy' but instead get the same jobs done in a pleasurable and light-hearted way. It really is a choice, and also a habit. When I decide to be a certain way, say lively and flirtatious, even if I'm at home by myself, I then get to practice it and it becomes more natural to me. Rechristen yourself as a lady of feminine charm and watch your experience *blossom*.

33. **Reframe 'healthy' as 'the good life'**. I remember meeting a lovely couple at a dinner through work friends; they grew up in New Zealand but the husband had Italian heritage. They both talked about how they choose to live the European way, following his family culture from the old country. At dinner, which was just a casual barbeque, his wife contributed the

biggest and most lush salad I have ever seen. It was amazingly delicious and looked incredible layered in a big glass bowl; the type of salad where there were lots of unexpected ingredients and it was a main component of the meal rather than an obligatory few leaves on the side of your plate. You could tell this was part of her repertoire when really, most people I know don't eat salads a lot. I heard them both talking to people about enjoying good food; clearly they valued their health and enjoyed high-quality natural foods. Do this for yourself; make being healthy a preference and your key to *la dolce vita*.

34. **Say *non* to snacking and drinking**. Unless it's at dinner when you might have a glass of wine or sparkling water by your plate, keep your food and drink separate. Don't eat when you have a coffee or cold drink. I wanted to do this, but it was hard at first. I associated my mid-morning *cafe au lait* with a muffin or something similar. Now I don't even think about eating anything, the coffee is enough. It was the same with my *aperitivo* (happy hour) drink before dinner. I couldn't *not* have potato chips, and then one day, I just... didn't, and never looked back. It was a simple decision to become a non-snacking lady and I felt so much more elegant as a result. And it was far easier to keep a stable weight too.

35. **Collect chic sightings**. Many years ago, I belonged to an online French Chic forum where ladies like myself would come together and report on fun plans, dreamy goals and talk about food, fashion and being their best, all through a Francophile lens. Frequently someone would report a 'chic sighting' – someone they had seen who inspired them. Their outfit would be described, where they were, and what action the person had inspired in them. The French Chic forum is long gone, but you can collect chic sightings for your own inspiration. Dedicate a notebook to this and it will be fun to jot them down and read them back too. Write down the date and place, a brief description of the person, and what it was that inspired you most. For example, it might be someone's bright silky scarf tied around their handbag or an outfit all in shades of white and cream. Or perhaps their beautiful posture, confident demeanour, or the fact that they were laughing unselfconsciously with their friend. My notebook for chic sightings is a document on my computer and while it is not added to often, I have had it for a long time and when I read through it every now and again, I can instantly picture the person I was inspired by. It is a valuable, personalized resource to help keep your standards high, and inspire you to try new things as well as always be your best.

36. **Add fun trends to your style**. Euro style is quite classic but it is also light-hearted, making the most of quirky details. I like to keep my clothing choices simple, but then add something a little outrageous, such as my black-and-white houndstooth coat, or a new cross-body bag style with the thick woven strap. It is enjoyable (and financially savvy) to weave the latest trends into your style in little ways. And, if something really rings your bell and you do want to invest in it, your personal style is instantly elevated. It's not just a trend, it's something you would love anyway. I love the current fashion of wearing a bum bag (fanny pack) like a cross body bag. I haven't done it myself yet but I think it looks great!

37. **Entertain your friends** with home-cooked food and good wine. There is something so much more special about hosting people at home rather than going out. It's more personal, and you can set the scene with tons of candles, sultry music, and simple food. You can make some parts of the meal and buy other parts ready-made. It doesn't matter if you don't have a lot of room either. Think of those cozy restaurants where people are crammed in and they're having a great time. If your table seats six and you have ten around it, make *that* the vibe. Dim the lights, wear your highest heels (you don't have to walk far) and enjoy the

evening.

38. **Feel sensual in your skin**. One thing I love about the idealistic French or Italian lady is her sexiness – she is insouciant and carefree. Coming from sensible English and Scottish heritage and growing up in practical New Zealand, it's easy for me to forget about sexiness and sensuality as a state of mind. In some cultures playful flirtation is a way of life, and I so envy them for that! An Italian woman I met a few times through work several years ago was very warm and nurturing at the same time as being sexy in that uniquely Italian way, good fun and also a good conversationalist. She would touch my arm or shoulder often while talking in the office, and kissed me on the cheek (just the one, not a double kiss) when she arrived and left. This was in a work environment and it felt totally appropriate. This is the kind of sexiness I am talking about and who wouldn't want more of that? We can all invite a little more playfulness into our interactions, in a way that is comfortable to us of course. And it all starts with how we feel *in ourselves*.

39. **Live richer than your budget**. Something Europeans are renowned for is living a life full of richness. We can do this too, by valuing experiences over possessions, living in a home

that is the right size for us, enjoying the clothes we already own instead of shopping for more, choosing free leisure activities such as people-watching outside a café or bar, reading a book in the park, visiting friends or inviting them over, being a *flâneur* around town (a *flâneur* is someone who enjoys strolling the city or their surroundings as a way to relax and observe), having hobbies and pastimes other than shopping, and insourcing services that we might otherwise outsource. I love seeing how thrifty I can be at the same time as living a fabulous life. It's so fun.

40. **Simplify your drinks menu**. It feels more European to drink only beer, wine or water – I don't find soft drink elegant in the least! Cocktails are very Euro-style too – think an Aperol Spritz in the summer or a fashionable Negroni. In my ideal European-inspired fridge, I would have sparkling and still water along with different wines, and some beer for my husband. With regards to hot drinks, apparently it's not the done thing to drink milky coffees after lunch; they are a morning beverage only. Black coffee always feels *très* stylish though, so why not learn to appreciate that?

41. **Cultivate your mystique**. Talking less in any situation is *the best* way to cultivate

mystique. Keep private information to yourself and try never to have to say the words, 'Sorry, TMI' ('too much information') after a conversation with someone. Move in silence. These are all reminders I tell myself often since I come from a genetic background of talkers. There is *a lot of talking* in my family I tell you. So if you too feel that you sometimes have a mouth like a torn sack (such a funny saying but also mortifying if the one they are talking about is you), take this to heart. Let people wonder what you might whisper next, rather than try to get away from you to halt the flow of words.

42. **Play French music at home**, both old and new to keep that feeling of French charm and lightness within you. Or feel emboldened and *Italian Chic* with opera. I am not an opera purist; I like enjoyable background opera, not blow-your-socks off powerful voices. I know this sounds terrible, but that's okay, I'm good with being basic. Soundtracks from movies often provide good listenable music, and Woody Allen's *Match Point* movie album does this with opera. His *Midnight in Paris* album is also wonderful, as is *To Rome with Love*. In fact, you can't go wrong with a Woody Allen soundtrack. He is a strange man, but genius when it comes to choosing music to evoke emotion and style.

43. **Change how you think about food**.
Rather than only considering what is
convenient and tastes good, start to learn more
about what you put into your body. I know for
myself that it's often a bothersome chore to
cook dinner at night and sometimes I can
really resent it. If you feel the same, the
dreaded dinner time malaise can be alleviated
by doing your food prep in the morning or even
the night before, but also by how you view the
process of cooking and eating. Instead of being
annoyed that you have to cook again, make a
conscious decision that it is something you
enjoy doing for yourself and nourishing your
body with. It is worth spending time and
money on maintaining your body well because
it will be with you all your life. With this
mental switch, cooking gets to be a pleasure
and not an annoying task.

44. **Try different makeup looks**. Use the
tiniest amount of foundation, just enough to
even out your skin tone, and then spend more
time on your eye makeup. One day I observed
the makeup of an Italian colleague of mine –
she wore a creamy skin-tone base, eyeliner top
and bottom in a dark, dark teal with plenty of
mascara, and nude-tone lipstick (with visible
liner). I'm not so sure about the visible lipliner
look for me, but I do love the made-up-
eyes/natural lip combo. It's especially

flattering for us *femmes d'un certain âge* ('ladies of a certain age', i.e. older!) because not only does this look draw attention away from the lines above our top lip, but it plays up our eyes, which can require a little more help over time. Keeping the foundation base light is what keeps this makeup look fresh. Search online for 'Italian woman makeup' or 'French girl makeup' for a visual.

45. **Stock your *euro-chic* kitchen**. Don't keep food in the house that the 'French you' would not have around. Would she nibble on potato chips? *Non*! Would she put out a small wedge of camembert or little bowl of olives? Much better. I always feel chicer when I pour a glass of sparkling water in preference to soda or choose fresh fruit with Greek yoghurt instead of breakfast cereal. There are lots of little switches you can make in your diet that not only feel more stylish but will likely be healthier too. I'm not a fan of wasting food, so if I see something in my fridge, freezer, or pantry that the French Fiona would not buy I'll commit to not replacing it. And when I am at the supermarket, I will let my inner euro-chic girl fill the cart.

46. **Be her today – *act as if***. To put a spring in your step, imagine your name is Dominique and that you live in Paris. Pretend you are her

as you go throughout your day. Yes, this definitely qualifies for the 'delusional' category, but it's so much fun. Choose your favourite flavour (country) and a beautiful name for yourself, and then act as if you are her. You will find that you hold yourself taller and straighter, you are sultrier in your demeanour, and you will make different choices, *without effort* (which is the best part). Embody her. Become her. In Hollywood this is called method acting, so it comes with good credentials.

47. **Don't be afraid to stand out where you live**. You may be hesitant to really let your French or Italian self shine because of the people around you. Perhaps, like me, you live where it's normal to dress casual at best and there might only be a small pool of well-dressed people. But so what? Why not be part of their crowd instead of joining the masses? Let your light shine as you show up exactly how you want to. Inspire others by your example. I have heard many stories of ladies who dressed up and were complimented (and even thanked) by others. Practice your new makeup look with bombshell eyes. Blow-dry your hair to perfection. Wear your new jeans and pretty top even though you're only running errands. Make daily life your runway; imagine if the paparazzi were photographing

your everyday look for your fans – give them something to look at!

48. **Work to live**. You may have heard the saying, 'work to live, not live to work', which means you don't let your career or job be the most important thing in your life. Sure, do a good job, turn up on time, and be pleasant while you're there, but *put your real life first*. There is no prize at the end of your life for being the most dedicated employee. Most jobs would replace you instantly if you left, so why do you tie yourself up into knots over every little thing? Work is a means to make money so you can live your life. That's all. Lessen your attachment to your job. Train yourself not to think of it after hours. Your boss can have you while you're there, but not in the evenings or weekends. That's *your* time, and the separation is a necessary part of having good mental health. I know it's hard when there is pressure, but if you start with something small people will realize they don't own 'all' of you, just the part when you are at work.

49. **Adopt a '*So What?*' attitude to life**. You may have heard of 'the gallic shrug', a particularly French way of answering something they don't feel is anything to do with them. And the subtext is 'Not my problem'. So many of us take on everyone

else's burdens and end up feeling resentful and burnt out. You don't need to become cold and uncaring, but why not decide to become a self-possessed woman who lets others be who they are and stays in her own lane? 'So what' is a reminder for you to lead your own happy life. Not everything needs to be fixed by you. And you get to enjoy your life without taking on everyone else's problems. For those of us who are always running (unbidden) to the rescue of others, it's a way of being we might never have considered (that's how it felt for me when I first started practicing it). And the best part of all is that you give others the chance to strengthen their own self by having to step up to the plate. Tough love is not for you, it is to grow the other person.

50. **Be selective with your time, money, and energy**. You don't have to say yes to everything, whether it's big or small. You can take a moment to think, 'Do I really want to do this?' and then decide. It's easier to go with the flow, but when we start deciding for ourselves what we want, something shifts. Being intentional helps us step into our ideal life, helps us make our ideal life our real life. If we are sitting in a rowboat bobbing around we are going to end up in any old place, but if we steer that boat, we get to where we want to go. Starting to be more mindful of where we spend

our time and money is a great way to begin.

51. **Stop waiting**. Life is passing us by one second at a time, and if we are always waiting for 'something to happen' or our dream life to begin, we'll die one day having led a very unfulfilled life. Take pleasure in your existence now. You can decide to be happy right now and if you're not, do something about it. Ask yourself: '*Who do I want to be in my home or my environment? How do I want to spend my days? How do I want to show up in the world and express my personal style? How do I want to dine?*' Start to make small changes towards the life you've always wanted. *Wait no more.* Something that I am putting my foot on the gas about is having a more minimal home. I've always been drawn to this aesthetic and way of living, and recently I have been inspired to make it happen. Not overnight, but I am taking small steps every week towards this goal by decluttering more, buying less, and being intentional. I have also been keeping my head in the zone by surrounding myself with like-minded inspiration online so that I don't 'forget' and become like a normal person with a house full of clutter again (a.k.a. the old me.). What are you waiting for and how can you make a start on it today?

52. **Embrace your uniqueness and quirks**.
Imagine the you that you would be if you lived
in Paris, in your beautiful stone apartment. As
you strolled around the beautiful city, would
you say to yourself, 'Oh I really wish I looked
like her' or, 'I might copy that outfit'? *Non*, the
European you would be thinking about what
suits *her* unique personality, *her* colouring,
her body type, and *her* facial structure in terms
of how she does her eye makeup. She would be
looking at things that make *her* happy, and
embraces her uniqueness rather than trying to
be just like everyone else. *And* if she is inspired
by somebody, whether she knows them in real
life, or they are a celebrity, it is more about
taking the essence or a detail that sparks an
interest in her rather than copying their look
exactly. Be that confident girl. Take what you
consider to be your weaknesses and look at
them instead as your strengths. Play them up
and be the best version of *you*.

53. **Get yourself out of debt**. Europeans
famously live a less indebted life than those of
us in English-speaking countries. They will
save up and go without until they can afford
something (and not upgrade so often either).
They will have fewer possessions overall (their
smaller apartments help with this; there is
simply not the room). And they buy better but
less, instead of the bargain shopping mentality

which I know I have been sucked into on many occasions. From today, make getting out of debt your highest goal. *You have so many more options without debt.* For a start, do not go into any new debt. Then, start paying off your loans beginning with consumer debt: credit cards and personal loans. Then your car, and when you are down to the mortgage on your house, focus on that. I am not a financial advisor and this is not financial advice; it's just how I did it. Living with loans to pay off is stressful, and when I decided to become debt free my everyday life got better and better. These days my husband and I have no debt and only a very small mortgage which will be gone within two years. And we are 51 and 52 years old currently. We have never had astronomical incomes; we just kept our 'eyes on the prize' and made life fabulous without spending a lot of money. It can be done, and if you make it a fun game you will never feel like you are 'cutting back'.

54. **Develop a sense of charm**. Make progress on your plans and dreams without feeling the need to update everyone that you come across. Keep most of your thoughts in your secret garden and only share your deepest feelings and vulnerabilities with one or two people close to you whom you can trust. Smile and say 'Thank you' when someone compliments you

instead of deflecting their words of praise or trying to downplay them. Communicate in other ways than speaking i.e. warm eye contact, a light touch on the arm or hand, open body language (shoulders back and arms down rather than folded), and lightly expressive hand movements. Become that lady who others are drawn to her aura.

55. **Create your *haute couture* mindset**. In the tradition of the great Parisian ateliers, piece together your ideal life with exquisite hand stitches. *Haute couture* is 'the creation of impeccable, custom-fitted high-end garments often utilizing handmade, one-of-a-kind embellishments'. Imagine a life like that: custom-fitted, high-end, and one-of-a-kind. Start with your mind, by developing it into your greatest asset. Of any decision, ask yourself if it is leading you towards your *haute couture* life or away from it? Is that decision worthy of your bespoke, high-end way of living? It doesn't matter whether your ideal life is top shelf expensive, or exquisite in its simplicity. It all starts from the same focused mindset. *Become bespoke.*

56. **Read the books you own**. Do you have books on your shelf at home (whether on your Kindle or actual paper books) that you want to read and have been meaning to read but still

have not opened them no matter how tempting the story or topic? Yeah, me too, and it's because screens get in the way. Let's start by choosing one book and committing to reading it. And if you don't want to read it given the (gentle) ultimatum? Put it in your donation box. Go through your books in this way and gain the value – and inspiration or entertainment – from books you already own; before you buy more, and before you go to scroll Twitter. Be a person who reads, who participates in her home environment and actually enjoys the items she has collected.

57. **Indulge in your favourite cliches**. My French-inspired life is so cliched, and I love it. I've planted red-orange geraniums in the garden, I make myself a café crème with my Nespresso machine each morning, and I adore playing French or Italian music as a delightful background detail at home. I wear scarves, perfume, and bright lipstick sometimes. I have a small collection of ballet flats, and a striped *bateau*-neck top is always a classic to me. Incorporate into your life all the things you know are total cliches in the French Chic (or Italian Chic or... Choose Your Chic) style but you love them anyway. And you don't have to do all these things forever either. I used to love wearing a beret in the winter and saying a cheery 'Bonjour' to people, but I don't

anymore. I just go with the flow of what feels good at the time. It doesn't matter what people think, as long as *you are happy* and you do what inspires *you*.

58. **Knit, crochet or sew** – be creative. Having a handcraft prevents mindless snacking as you can't knit or do needlepoint if your hands are sticky from chocolate, or greasy from potato chips. I always like to keep my hands busy when I am watching tv or a movie so try to keep a portable project by the sofa. I also keep my sewing desk tidy most of the time so it is inviting when I feel like being creative or need to hem a pair of trousers. I always feel more chic when I sew or knit and create (especially if I follow a pattern from German fashion sewing magazine *Burda Style*). I imagine my French self creating her own designer pieces on a tiny sewing machine in the corner of her apartment in Paris!

59. **Focus on one small habit each week**. In creating your European style life, there will be lots of fun tweaks to bring into your orbit. Give yourself the best chance of success by working on them one at a time. Write everything down you want to do, and choose one to focus on each week. You might decide to do 'no snacking' the first week, making sure your meals are filling and with enough protein to

get you through to your next meal without becoming hungry. Enjoyable upgrades for other weeks might be keeping good posture, accessorizing your outfits more, doing your makeup differently, eating fresh fruit after each meal, or moisturizing your whole body daily. You might even carry on the previous week's habit while you add the next one.

60. **Consider your 'signature look'**. Many stylish women are instantly recognizable because their outfits – even on different days – have a similarity about them. These well-dressed ladies have curated their best look and made it into a sort of uniform whether intentionally or unintentionally. Some take it to minimalist extremes, and for others it's that they have found the most flattering silhouette for their body type and recreate it with different fabrics and colours, casual or dressy. Take the time to look at what outfits make you feel your best and wear them more, as well as keeping your ideal look in mind when you shop.

61. **Dump the frump**. For some reason, I always end up with a few frumpy pieces in my closet. I love being comfortable so you think it would be that, but I have items that I feel fabulous in that are very comfortable too. No, it's when they are perhaps not quite the right shade of a

colour or the style isn't so modern. But still, I persist on holding onto these clothing items and wearing them, because there is not anything technically wrong with them. But what I do know is that I feel frumpy when I wear them. So, I am being strong and putting those pieces aside to donate. I know my closet and my style feels a million times better when I do that. If this is you too, please join me in *dumping the frump.* Just because we are all getting older each year doesn't mean we need to descend into clothing styles that make us feel older than we are. And I see plenty of ladies in their seventies, eighties and even nineties who are the opposite of frumpy, so it doesn't need to be a given as you age.

62. **Be organized for serenity**. Deciding to become an organized person isn't just about being efficient, it is about enjoying your life more. When you spend a little time each week ensuring that your home is decluttered, tidy, and all your possessions have a place to live, you will feel calmer and more peaceful. You will have less frown lines than someone who is constantly irritated by their messy home where they cannot find their car keys. It's not lazy to want a serene and peaceful life, it's just smart. You are allowed to enjoy yourself while you live your life. It's not meant to be a burdensome uphill battle every day! Pare

down your belongings, simplify your schedule, do tasks as quickly as you can (no multi-tasking!) and always ask yourself, 'How can I make this easier?'

63. **Serve your meals in courses**. Instead of piling everything onto one plate, why not try dining in courses the European way? Serve your side salad in a bowl next to your dinner plate. Have a dish of sliced fruit for afters. Maybe a cheese selection. Leave time between each course and enjoy being at the table and chatting. If your family vacuum everything down, bring the plates out from the kitchen one at a time. Get them used to spending more than seven minutes at the dining table, or even eating at the dining table at all. You might not be able to swing it every night, but try it on the weekend and then gradually introduce one or two more nights during the week. My mother always tried to make my siblings and me less like savages at the table and I thank her for that. She loves to make soup and is very good at it, so she would always start with a soup course, then our lunch or dinner, and sometimes a pudding too. Thanks mum!

64. **Study the arts**. Choose something you are interested in such as art history, English literature, or medieval music. Search out documentaries, books, and online sources to

learn more. Broaden your scope from only watching current affairs and popular culture. What is most fascinating about studying 'old things' is that it makes you realize how much was already happening hundreds, sometimes thousands of years before you were born. It can really boggle the mind (in a good way). This helps you be less focused on the minutiae, and more on the big picture, other people, and other cultures. At the very least, you will have a deep appreciation in the beauty of what you are studying. Plus, it asks of you to contemplate just what *you* are going to contribute to the world for future generations to value!

65. **Learn how to make an omelette**. For a quick, easy, and delicious lunch for one, I often make myself scrambled eggs or an omelette. Imagine having *omelette aux fines herbes* as one of your signature dishes that you have perfected and can whip up in an instant? There are plenty of recipes and videos online; Julia Child is inspiring to watch. You can keep it simple with fresh herbs and a little cheese, or use up food you have in the fridge. A few mushrooms, even one, sliced finely is plenty. Leftover salami. Finely diced capsicum (bell pepper) is a favourite for me. And while you're at it, learn how to crack eggs with one hand. Gordon Ramsay 'taught' me (in a video) once,

and I've never gone back. It's actually very easy and people are so impressed when you do it!

66. **Know the basics of homekeeping**. Maybe you desire a more independent life than being a wife and/or mother, or maybe you are both of those things and have vowed never to cook a meal. I believe we all get to choose what we want to do. However, it is a valuable skill to be able to run a home, even if you choose to outsource a lot of tasks, or lead a very simple and minimal life by yourself. It's just part of being a grown-up when you know your bills are paid on time, your pantry is organized, and that the behind-the-scenes of your life is ticking over neatly. It might be cool to float through life with an unhurried, insouciant air, but you need a solid foundation; that practical streak so you know how to cook yourself a meal or where to turn the water off on your property. I am always of the opinion that the perfect way to live is a combination of having your head in the clouds and feet firmly on the ground.

67. **Redefine your life periodically**. One year can roll into the next, and even though we might make new year's resolutions and plans and goals for ourselves, do many of us often consider the big picture? It's a good idea to take stock of where you are at and what you

have achieved. Not just work-wise, but are you happy with all aspects of your life? Is there any part of it that is not up to par? When you take a moment to look at your life as a whole, you can see where you are being held back and work on elevating that category. Where are you winning, and where are you letting yourself down? Then, ask yourself how your chic, next-level self would deal with any area that is not as good as you'd like. Would she make one big change that sweeps through and upgrades everything in a single swoop? Or does she feel more comfortable with micro-changes to her habits and her schedule that will effortlessly uplevel her experience? I prefer the latter, it just feels easier to me. But sometimes I am drawn to the first scenario. Both are valid, just start by pondering where you're at in life.

68. **Don't feel that you must slavishly copy** everything about a culture to be inspired by it. Each country and its people has its own good and not-so-good points. And you don't have to be like anybody else apart from yourself. But it's fun to get ideas and inspiration of different ways to be, ways that we might never have come across before in our own heritage and how we grew up. Finding your authentic self is one part where you were born and the family who raised you, one part your current environment, and the final part: *who you*

desire to be. Whatever rings your bell with happiness, follow that. Take the good points from cultures you are drawn to and infuse those ideas into how you live where you are. This is how you will create your most beautiful and inspired life.

69. **Create your own chic mentor** by giving yourself a new name. She will be a sort of muse for you as you make small changes to make your life more as you dream it could be. I have always liked the name Sabine as my chic muse. I imagine I am her as I choose what to wear for the day, or what to order at lunchtime. I don't even have to ask for her advice, she just gives it to me unsolicited! And always in a French accent too! And then sometimes I'll call on my Italian muse; she is more uninhibited, very earthy and sensual. I remember seeing a lady in Rome with wild curly blonde hair wearing a leather outfit in red, white and blue. It didn't look like a costume even though she was certainly eye-catching. I think it was just the way she liked to dress. I sometimes imagine her being my chic mentor and assisting me in being my most flamboyant self. Perhaps she can be Graziella. Where is your muse from and what are you going to call her?

70. **Don't be too 'put together' in your look**. This tip is a reminder for those of us who love

to look 'neat and tidy' (such as *moi*, and maybe you too) to be a little more undone when we dress. French ladies are famous for not looking too pristine. Their eyeliner may be artfully smudged; their hair flicky and a little messy looking; and their clothes not perfectly matched or styled. Yet they likely spent time in front of the mirror to look this way. Think 'messy with dressy' – it's a phrase I heard once and it goes well with the French girl aesthetic. Turn your cuffs back rather than roll and button them neatly. Show a peek of lacy camisole at the top of your blouse buttons. Never appear too studied and you will have cracked the code of French Chic!

71. **Dress with more dash than cash**. Study stylish people on how they put together expensive looking outfits and then learn to recreate your own version on a budget. I love to buy moderately-priced clothing and footwear, and pair them with a wow-factor accessory. This is how I feel happiest dressing. Or choose one or two trendy details from the current season and keep your look updated this way. It might be a hot colour that also happens to suit you, or a jeans finish or leg width. I love wearing skinny/fitted jeans for a clean silhouette but have just bought a pair of girlfriend jeans which I am enjoying playing around with to create different outfits.

72. **For the perfect 'Euro Chic' dinner**, pick up a piece of fresh white fish at the market to pan-fry in butter, adding a squeeze of lemon juice at the end. Plate with lightly steamed vegetables such as asparagus, green beans, or broccolini depending on the season, and dress your vegetables in a dash of olive oil. Serve with ground pepper and salt, and a glass of sparkling mineral water or a crisp Sauvignon Blanc (Sancerre). I promise, you will not only feel like you are dining in the south of France or Positano with your delicious supper, but you will have enjoyed a nutritious meal, *and* satiated yourself nicely. Bon appétit.

73. **Become proficient in scarf tying.** Knowing different ways to tie a scarf, whether it is around your neck, threaded through your belt loops or around a bag handle, will mark you as someone with European style. I have an Hermes pamphlet which shows simple ways to tie any scarf, and there are great YouTube videos which are sometimes easier to follow than written or illustrated instructions. If you are anything like me and have lovely scarves which you forget to wear, get them all out today and try a new technique. Scarves really are the perfect finishing touch to any outfit, but if you're like me, perhaps you just forget to wear them. Become known as the lady who always looks chic and put together via her

secret weapon – a scarf!

74. **Try a pared-down Euro-style wardrobe**.
Many homes in Europe are far smaller than in
other countries, and this applies to their
closets as well. Start to shop 'less but better'
(which doesn't always have to mean expensive;
for me 'better' means being more intentional
when I shop). Begin the process by putting
together a mix-and-match capsule wardrobe
just like the appealing visuals on Pinterest.
Curate yourself a 'perfect French wardrobe' for
a weekend away or just to wear over the next
few weeks at home. See how much easier it is
to dress yourself in the morning. I do my Euro-
style wardrobe with a few more clothes than
strict minimalists do, simply because I like the
variety. When I try to dress with a tiny number
of items, I become bored easily. But I certainly
have noticed how when I cleared out the pieces
which made me feel dowdy, frumpy, or guilty,
my closet was a much more inspiring place to
get dressed in. Play around with the right
amount of clothing for you.

75. **Know yourself and look your best**. The
true secret to 'French Chic' is to *be yourself*.
Wear what you love and build on that. It's a
balance between being inspired by others and
trying out different looks, but at your core
coming back to how you feel your best. And

this feeling will change over the course of your lifetime too. For a long time I wore soft tones and neutrals, but now I am attracted towards brighter colours and the blended tones don't feel so much like me anymore. I am also finding myself drawn to black after not desiring to wear it for many years. Always be asking yourself what you are guided towards by seeing how a colour or silhouette makes you feel. Feeling excited, optimistic, and sparkly are good indicators that these looks are the direction you want to go in, so give yourself permission to wear those clothes and be your most authentic self.

76. **Grow herbs at home**. Adding finishing touches to a meal in the form of chopped fresh parsley on scrambled eggs, stirring thyme into a creamy chicken sauce, or sprinkling rosemary sprigs into a big oven dish of roasted root vegetables as they cook will not only add to the flavour, but the look of your meal as well. And when you grow your own herbs there are a myriad of benefits: you will use them more often because they are right there ready to be snipped off (whether you have them just outside your kitchen in the garden or in pots), they will be fresher, they will be spray-free, and the cost is negligible since the little plants are not expensive. Your planter pots or kitchen garden will look *très chic* and European, and

there is the final bonus that all herbs have their own health benefits. Herbs are the bomb!

77. **Go to events**. If you don't look for them you will find that opportunities to do something different, socialize and get out and about can pass you by. A friend who works for the local inner city business association told me last week about an upcoming promotion. It is on for one night only and is called *La Passeggiata Cocktail Walk*. You get a little passport which lists the participating bars and cafes, and from 5pm to 8pm people dress up, stroll around, grab a drink and generally chit chat and be out to 'see and be seen', just like the Italian tradition of *passeggiata*. I am so excited for this! And equally, you will find art exhibitions, live acts in small venues, and local theatre if you seek them out. You get to support local initiatives, change your visual landscape, soak in new inspiration, and have a chance to wear your nice clothes. I *always* feel more European when I make an effort to participate in events that are on.

78. **Have your signature dishes**. Why not practice and become known for a few signature dishes? My mother has her shortbread and pavlova. My cousin Gareth does a Sunday dinner with extra crispy roast potatoes. And I love to make apple crumble in the winter. The

excellent thing about having your own signature dishes is that they are often the items on a menu you love most, so you always get to eat your favourite food. Think about what you most like to cook and eat, and do them often so you can prepare them without a recipe, and you know the timings as well. When you have a few signature dishes up your sleeve, you will also feel more confident inviting others around for a meal.

79. **Eliminate stress as much as possible**. This may just be in my imagination, but for me, my inner French or Italian girl does not rush about trying to do more than is humanly possible in one day. She does not get little pinched lines around her mouth because she is silently tut-tutting others like I used to. *Non*, she lives her life in a relaxed manner. She does one thing at a time. She gets ready in the morning in a leisurely fashion (and simplifies her beauty regime so it is not onerous). She gives herself the pleasure of daily reading time with a real book. She takes her makeup off after dinner and enjoys a relaxed prelude to bedtime. Her weekends are for strolls, cafes, and movies at the theatre. She has set her life up for leisure and play. Doesn't this all sound deliciously peaceful and comforting? And it is attainable, I promise. In your own way of course, but there is always something you can

do to lower your stress and make life more enjoyable. This is what motivates me to keep my life simple and my home decluttered. Maybe you too?

80. **Eliminate toxicity**. You will find it easier to lead a happier and more relaxed life if you identify toxic elements and rid yourself of them as much as possible. Don't keep doing things just because you feel guilty stopping, such as a volunteer position you have done for a long time, for example. If the stress is taking a toll on your wellbeing or your workload has increased, bow out. In addition, watch as little news as you can, preferably none. Or choose a news source that is not sensationalist and check in once a week. *Keep all toxic people away from you.* If you feel drained or bad after spending time with someone, reduce how often you see them or simply drift away. Life is too short, and it may even be shortened with exposure to drama and stress! When you identify and reduce toxicity as much as you can, your blood pressure will thank you, and you will find that life feels a little lighter. In my dealings with Europeans, they find it far easier to say what they want, to the point that it can seem abrupt to us people-pleasers from English-speaking countries. Change things as gently as you can, or with humour if that feels better, but *do it*.

81. **Value sleep**. Sleep is so underrated as a beauty and wellness essential. It seems 'boring' to go to bed early, but when you have a late night or broken sleep, you will know all about it. In the morning you look in the mirror and gasp at how haggard you look. It's horrifying! Long before plastic surgery and beauty treatments such as Botox, the French lady knew that a good night's sleep was the best thing you could do to give your skin a healthy glow. And it's valuable to your whole system because resting well means your body gets a chance to renew its cells while you sleep. I honestly don't know how Europeans can get enough sleep with their famous late mealtimes, because they still get up early. But I do know many have an afternoon siesta. I am not a daytime sleeper, so I choose, for the most part, to go to bed early. I also like to calm myself with a pleasant evening routine so that I can sleep well too (taking my time to wash my face and moisturize, reading a book etc).

82. **Get outside every day**. Instead of eating lunch at your desk, take it outside and eat at a park. If you're in the city, stroll around window shopping. If you work on an industrial estate there will still be somewhere to sit and soak in some Vitamin D. Or, have your own picnic rug in the car. If it's raining, take an umbrella and go for a fifteen-minute walk. Leave a pair of

sneakers under your desk or in your locker. If you work from home sip your coffee on the patio or balcony. No matter your situation, 'take the air' and get outside. You will connect with nature and feel rejuvenated. If you are in a busy environment, it's a chance to people watch too!

83. **Build your chic library**. I have a small collection of books on my shelf that I doubt will ever be decluttered. They bring me comfort and pleasure and lift me up when I need a boost. My favourite authors are Anne Barone, Mireille Guiliano, Jennifer L. Scott, Raeleen D'Agostino Mautner, Helena Frith Powell, Tish Jett, Pamela Druckerman, Debra Ollivier, and Jamie Cat Callan. E.J. Gore's 'French Lessons' also deserves a special mention. It is a delightful book. I have many of these authors both as eBooks and in print, because as much as I love to have them on my Kindle for instant access anywhere, I equally enjoy choosing a volume from my bookshelf in the hall for a few minutes of inspiration. Build up your library, whether they are eBooks, in print or both, then relax in comfort knowing they will always be there to support and uplift you.

84. **Design your own Euro-style menu plan**. I have never been one to write out a week's

worth of dinners and stick to the list religiously. It works better for me to plan two or three days ahead instead. But what does inspire me is to imagine what I would dine on if I was that chic lady living in Rome. What would she have in her fridge? Her pantry? What kinds of dinners would she put together? What would she have for lunch? Or for breakfast? Creating a menu for your ideal self is a fun angle to effortlessly upgrade your food choices. Not only do you get new ideas customized to your tastes, but you will find that packaged foods are less appealing and thus greatly minimized. No-one's ideal lady ever lies around emptying a large bag of potato chips into her mouth!

85. **Look presentable every day**. Coco Chanel said, 'I don't understand how a woman can leave the house without fixing herself up a little – if only out of politeness. And then, you never know, maybe that's the day she has a date with destiny.' Even if I am only going to the supermarket, I dress well now, but I can't say that was always the case. I can remember thinking, 'I'm only dashing in for a few things, I won't see anyone.' And of course, that's exactly when I *would* bump into somebody. If it becomes something you practice and then turns into a habit, there is no need to ask yourself whether you should do it or not; it's

just something you always do. And as Coco says, it is good manners to look nice. We do it not only for ourselves, but also because other people have eyes and it is more pleasant for them. This is what I read about Parisians – they dress well almost as a social service. I think this is a fabulous way to be!

86. **Never talk about dieting**. Let's say you decide your clothes are getting a little tight and want to do something about it. You might choose to try Intermittent Fasting, decide to cut back on sugar, alcohol, or bread (whatever your downfall is), or have smaller portions. No matter your style of 'cutting back', the key secret is that *you tell no-one*. It's just something you do for yourself and you keep it in your secret garden, with an excited butterfly feeling because you know you are going to feel better in yourself and look great in your clothes. Currently I am choosing to break my overnight fast at noon, because we eat dinner quite late. I have not mentioned this to my husband once, but I'm sure he has noticed. Unlike in the past, I have not made a grand proclamation that I am going to be healthier or snack less or eat more fruit. Your health plan will be easier to stick to when you resist the urge to share it with everyone, but it's good etiquette too – other people's diets are so boring. *Save your words, show them the*

results instead.

87. **'To thine own self be true'**. This line from William Shakespeare's 'Hamlet' is one of my favourite mottos and it fits perfectly with what I believe is the hidden secret within 'French Chic' or 'Italian Chic'. Yes, it's about looking stylish and having that European insouciance, but it's also about living a life which aligns with your true values. It's about letting pressure and expectations from others fall away, and not creating extra work which prevents you from living a low-stress life of utter joy and pleasure. Ponder this point and decide that you are going to cultivate your *joie de vivre* ('exuberant enjoyment of life') by being true to yourself in what you choose to wear, what activities you enjoy, and how you desire to live your life.

88. **Take time for yourself**. Many of us save our relaxing time for when we are on holiday. If we are at home we notice jobs that need to be completed and it's not easy to put our feet up. We feel lazy and cannot sit down until everything is done. And of course everything is *never* done. So another day goes by when we haven't participated in anything fun and restorative for ourselves. I am here to give you – and me – permission to have that mini-break *every single day*. Surely we all have time

for fifteen minutes? And could we work it up to half an hour or even an hour? What are you going to do in your relaxing time? You could garden, watch a movie, write something, sew or knit a little, read a great book, go to a concert or the theatre, window shop in town, have a coffee in a café, design, create, or do something outdoorsy or sporty. The list is long! Make your own notes on what would help your life feel more in vacation mode, and decide when in your day you are going to take some time for yourself.

89. **Decide to be unflappable always**. Have you ever come across someone who is serene and centred in a way that makes *you* feel calmer? I have found when I choose to be that undramatic person in my own life, it feels so good. When I drop something and break it, I can choose to simply clear it up and move on, or I can wail to myself how stupid I am and that it was my favourite mug and how could I have been so silly... It is not becoming, even if I am the only one viewing me. And it doesn't rewind time either. Unfortunately. The same goes in a serious situation. When you are drama-free and focused, you are much more effective. It really is a choice in any situation to deal with it or fall apart. Choose to remain grounded. The more you do this, the more it will be your natural state. You will make others

feel safer, feel better in yourself, and you will find you have less attachment to the past. Things happen all the time. How you deal with them is up to you.

90. **Know how to do a few kitchen staples well**. I used to buy all sorts of bottled salad dressings, and I still do keep a few on hand such as aioli or mayonnaise, but I mostly make my own dressings now – usually a simple vinaigrette comprised of olive oil and vinegar – red wine, white wine or balsamic. I prefer less vinegar and more oil, and I might grind some fresh pepper and salt on top too. There are wonderful traditional vinaigrette recipes online, including such ingredients as mustard, a whole garlic clove to flavour but not be eaten, and fresh herbs. It's nice to be able to make a two-ingredient vinaigrette just for one meal, or if I'm in a chef mood, to make a batch with a recipe.

91. **Be open to being more visible**. When you upgrade your standards on how you are going to be, particularly with clothing and grooming, you might feel a little uncomfortable, a little too 'extra' amongst the people you normally hang around with. A great piece of advice I heard made me feel okay with that. It was along the lines of: 'We're not trying to fit in, we're trying to stand out.' As in, we're not

trying to blend in with the crowd by dressing in a way that makes us feel comfortable (and invisible), we are happy to go with our own preferred level of style and let what happens, happen. Likely all that will happen is that you will be treated better. Remember that when you feel anxious that all eyes will be on you if you wear what you want to wear and do your hair and makeup, with polished nails. *You're not trying to fit in, you're trying to stand out*. And it can be standing out 5% or going all in. You get to choose. And, you might find others rising up too. Seeing you uplevel gives them the inspiration and permission to do the same.

92. **Be financially savvy**. A fun little game I like to play with myself is to see how little I can spend and still have that good feeling of wellbeing. When you do this, you will find unnecessary expenditures disappear and you likely won't even miss what you used to buy. Rather than frittering away your money on chocolate bars, coffee, and cheap tops, save it for what you would really love such as a high-quality item of clothing that you will wear for many years. Plus, you will be learning to embrace self-control and self-discipline in a way that perhaps you thought was never possible for you.

93. **Create your own sense of sanctuary at home** so you can go out and face the world each day with well-rested confidence. Imagine if you lived in a tiny and elegant apartment in the middle of your preferred European city. It would be your haven from a busy world. Somewhere you could return to each night after an invigorating day of being amazing. You would decorate it in a way that speaks to your soft heart, keep it clean and welcoming, and be thoughtful of the possessions you bring into it. There is no reason you can't bring the essence of this vision right here to your current life at home. Treat where you live as your peaceful refuge, your inspiring shelter, and care for and curate it to be everything you need.

94. **Find a place of peace within your home**. And, to take things one step further, create an actual European-inspired nook somewhere just for you. It might be a small library area with all your favourite inspiration, a comfy chair with a small table and your current reading material. Or an *haute couture* fashion area in your wardrobe, complete with runway images that make you happy. Maybe it's the feeling of a Parisian *parfumier* in your bathroom with touches of pink and gold, or the ambience of a high-end spa where you do your facial therapies. Whatever your vision is, find

a small (or big) way to bring it into your home.

95. **Walk more where you live**. Go window-shopping in town, or for a stroll on your lunch break. Walk through a park on the weekend, not just for 'exercise' but because it's pleasurable to take in nature and stretch your legs. Whenever I walk, I feel very European, whether it's an exercise walk near home, or driving to the nearby waterfront or a public park to meander around on a sunny weekend afternoon. Sometimes I'll park my car in town and walk to do all my errands rather than move my car to each place. Of course, time available and demands such an item that you are picking up being large will dictate if this is practicable, but if you can walk more, you can infuse that European habit of walking places into your everyday. This is how Europeans on the whole stay slimmer than their counterparts in other countries – they are less sedentary.

96. **Celebrate family moments**. I love to host 'big family dinners' every so often; mostly they will be for someone's birthday, a special event such as Easter, Christmas, or a long weekend, or to welcome family members who are in town. It's easy to let occasions pass without marking them, and it's just as easy to host a simple and fun affair. I have always coveted

the 'Italian long lunch' at an outdoor table. I haven't managed the outdoor bit yet, but I do love a long table with all my family around eating, drinking, joking, and laughing. If necessary, I'll place a second table at the end of our dining table to elongate it and put two white tablecloths over them. I clear the room and place this extra-long table as the showpiece in the centre of the room. It is such a jovial occasion and everyone appreciates the get-together.

97. **Eliminate most sugar from your life**. One thing I have noticed in my study of the French or Italian woman is that she eats far less sugar than me. She will have tiny amounts at appropriate times, but even the sweet treats she eats will be low in sugar, such as dark chocolate, a tiny and rich chocolate mousse, or fresh berries and whipped cream. And there is frequency too. A lady I came across on Instagram who had lived in Paris for many years posted a picture of the fruit custard tart from a café that she said was her favourite treat. I left a comment and asked how often she would have one. She kindly responded and said 'about once a month'. This gave me a new insight in that, even if I chose to eat healthy and be low-sugar, it wouldn't mean no treats ever again. And I can imagine you would enjoy that café sweet even more if you didn't have it

every day or even every week.

98. **What does your Inner French Girl want to do today**? What deserves your 100% priority? It doesn't matter whether your day is a workday, weekend, or vacation. As you are reading this book, what is she asking of you? Does she want you to play more and feel lighter in spirit? Does she want you to provide her with nourishing food that will bring her beauty, health, and satisfaction? Does she want you to amp up your personal style today, putting on a different pair of earrings and spritzing your wrists with your 'best' perfume even if you're only going to work? Ask your inner French (or Italian, or Spanish, whoever you prefer) girl every day what she needs and let her guide you.

99. **Unbutton your sensuality**. European women are more passionate than many of us more practical souls. Passionate in the relationship sense, and also in the way they live their life. I know I am romanticizing European women here – I see that – but it's a lovely reminder for me, and for you too if you like. Take life less seriously, literally unbutton your shirt one more and let your lacy camisole show, dance through your day. Be that insouciant, unbothered, charismatic lady. You can still be your orderly, sensible self, but a

sprinkling of Italian fairy dust to loosen up and soften the face never hurt anyone!

100. **Radiate confidence**. The Parisian lady feels positive about her looks and her body, no matter that she is nowhere near perfect. She feels assured in her home and her entertaining style. She has faith in how she loves and is loved back. You can see all this in the way she walks, and with her speech and her demeanour. She never second-guesses herself and she trusts herself implicitly. Imagine if you adopted supreme belief in yourself, that you were always doing the right thing and moved through the world from that place? Start being your most confident and optimistic self today, try it on and see how it feels. I like it on you, in fact it really suits you!

And there we have it. One hundred ways to live your life with a European sensibility. Now I hand the keys to Versailles over to you. Saunter on, keep going. Have fun dreaming up your most fabulous European inspired life and implementing small changes as you feel called to.

There is no 'work to do', it's all good. Let yourself feel light and easy. Float above the ground. Know that your life will become better and better each year, even though you are getting older. You're just getting started! *Each year will outshine the last.* Since I borrowed this thought from Louise Hay, it has been that way for me and I know it will be the same for you.

And to finish, please enjoy this extra bonus... (because I can never help myself – I especially love an inspiring list to send you off with). Read on!

50 more ways to
bring a little European flair
into your life

1. Create your own inspiration piece about your 'Italian life' or your 'French life' in a journal. Note down ideas of how you would be if you **infused the essence of that style** into your life, every day.

2. **Peruse French bistro menus** online (I zoom into photos to read what is written on the blackboard) to get ideas for a stylish, yet simple meal. Perhaps *bœuf bourguignon* and a glass of red wine for dinner tonight?

3. Try a different lipstick. Mostly I wear a pinky-bronze lipstick lightly applied with gloss on top, but sometimes I'll choose a vibrant matte red or hot pink shade instead and it feels so good. You

will likely already own **a lipstick which is 'a bit much'** so you don't reach for it very often, but just for today, go for it!

4. Ask your **French or Italian alter ego to help you out** in any situation whether it is a wardrobe dilemma or relationship issue. 'She' could be the one giving you guidance. When I have tried this she is actually very wise, and I have been given excellent advice.

5. **Embody the spirit of elegance** wherever you can. The definition of elegance talks of effectiveness, neatness, and simplicity. Pare down to a chic lifestyle by cleaning out what you can, whether it is a habit, clutter in your home, or a seasonal update to your personal style.

6. Be active every day. Go for a twenty-minute walk. Vacuum the house. Do some decluttering and organizing. Window shop. When you find that you've been sitting for a while, get up and do something. Even in an office situation this is doable. **Always be moving**.

7. 'Book in' spa time once a week. Exfoliate your face and apply a mask before bed to **pamper your complexion** and unwind from the day. Sip herbal tea and read a book while you wait for your mask to work.

8. Look at each day as another **chance to be your best European-inspired self** – how you dress appropriate to what you are doing, how you dine, what you read, who you converse with, and the activities you partake in.

9. Choose the **healthiest option in any situation** you find yourself in. You can't always control the food choices, say if you're meeting a friend at a café, but you can make the best choice from their selection. It's a nice way of balance that promotes long-term vitality without being too strict on yourself.

10. When you are inspired to add a detail to your look (such as building a monochrome outfit, wearing a scarf, or changing your lipstick colour), or practice a certain way of being (perhaps talking less and having mystique) do it straight away. **Apply yourself, don't just think about it**. Embodying your inspiration is far better than simply reading, thinking, and dreaming about it. This is how you will bring your idealistic French girl into your real life.

11. Tidy and **display your accessories** in your closet so you reach for them more often. 'Out of sight, out of mind' is how I keep forgetting to wear a scarf or change out my handbag!

12. Make **a list of things you enjoy doing** and ensure you *do them*. For me, it's reading, daydreaming, stretching, being creative, sewing, and making my home as beautiful as I can by tidying, rearranging, and creating ambience with music, candles, and décor.

13. **Add cell-plumping fat to your meals**. A small amount of real butter, a few slices of avocado, dressing salad leaves with a dash of olive oil, eating raw nuts, or pouring cream or whole milk into your coffee are all delicious ways of adding fat to your meals. Fat makes everything taste better! And 'good' fats are great for your skin as well as keeping you satiated between meals.

14. Make **a conscious decision on how you are going to live**, and then embody that, daily. Write a little note to remind yourself of your desires, on the inside cover of your planner, as a note on your phone, or tuck a slip of paper into your wallet.

15. Each day this week, **add one extra touch** to your outfit. Feel pretty and creative by adding a scarf, wearing different earrings than usual, or layering a blazer more for fashion than the weather.

16. Prioritize **beauty, quality, and style**, even in the most routine aspects of your daily life. When you take care of the little things you will see your enjoyment blossom.

17. Transform an ordinary day by looking at everything as an **opportunity to please your senses** just like *Amelie* did in her self-titled movie. As you chop vegetables for dinner gaze in wonder at the rich shades Mother Nature provided for your nourishment and enjoyment. Smooth your hands over the fabric of a top and appreciate the fine weave as you hang it up. Breathe in that unique smell which arises just as the rain starts in summer. There is beauty for the senses everywhere when you look for it.

18. Choose **simplicity as a way of life**. The opposite, of course, is complication, which doesn't sound nearly as nice, does it? Remove distractions to ensure you have time to enjoy what is important to you.

19. No matter your stage of life, **slow down**. Be less hurried, more present. Prove to yourself that you will get just as much done and with more pleasure too when you choose not to be flustered or chaotic.

20. Research **a small list of easy-to-make snacks** or small meals that you enjoy, so you

will never find yourself stuck in a drive-thru because you forgot to think ahead.

21. Employ **European self-discipline** – discipline in how you eat, how you care for yourself, and with money. But rather than think of it as deprivation, flip it around to see that you are giving yourself *the world* when you practice being a self-disciplined lady. It will put you on the path to receiving everything you ever wanted.

22. Dress and groom yourself **to the best of your ability**, no matter your age, height, weight, or monetary situation. We can all do our best with what we have.

23. Hang **your clothes on the same type of hanger**, or perhaps two types such as white wooden for tops, and white felt for bottoms. Use what you have and go for a uniformity. It makes such a difference and feels like you are shopping in your own boutique when all the hangers match. And if you find yourself a hanger or two short, why not declutter that number of items?

24. **Learn a few words of your favourite language**. It's hard to completely learn a language unless you are living in that country and have a chance to use it daily, but even a few words feels good. My dog groomer is from

Milan, so I always say *Buongiorno* or *Grazie* to her.

25. **Set boundaries and practice tough love**. Unless you have a child under the age of eighteen, you are only responsible for yourself. You do not need to bail anybody out, prop them up, or exhaust yourself looking after them. Give others the gift of the chance to take care of themselves. It will grow them and be for their benefit, *and* lessen the burden on you.

26. **Design your own '52 weeks to chic' plan**, by dreaming up fifty-two changes, improvements, or desires that you'd love to bring into your life. Focus on one each week and look forward to a fabulous 'new you' in a year's time!

27. Don't worry about everything you did or didn't do in the past or what the future might bring, just focus on where you are right now and **make the most of *this* time**. Practice living in the present.

28. **Always wear earrings**. Even if you are not going anywhere, always have earrings on. They just add a little something, without any effort apart from putting them on in the morning. Pearl or 'diamond' studs are my go-to; they look pretty and I don't have to worry about them

catching on anything.

29. If anyone ever says anything unkind, know that it is all about them and never about you. **Don't take things personally**, and instead stay in your lane, being you. Smile and thank them. *Thank them for showing their true self.*

30. **Declutter for your dream life**. Pretend you are moving to Paris, or any other city that occupies your dreams, and eliminate anything you would not furnish your beautiful Parisian apartment with.

31. Just for one day, or even one hour, **imagine you are being filmed**. You are in the movie of your life! See how this awareness affects your movements, how you dress, and what you eat. Even the tone of your voice may change. When I am 'on film', I move with exquisite grace and intention.

32. **Go beyond** fashion by cultivating your own personal style, and accessorize with grace and poise. Include everything around you – how you keep your car, your home, and your demeanour.

33. Identify what items in your home enhance your life, what are just there because they've always been there, and what deplete your energy. Make plans to rid yourself of the energy depleters, rejoice in the enhancers, and put the rest on

probation. **Have regular cleanouts**.

34. **Embrace getting older**. In Europe, older women are cherished, and it shows in their confidence. Be that lady in her fifties rocking a bikini on the beach. Be fabulous and love *the power of being you*.

35. Look slimmer and taller instantly **by keeping good posture**. Pull your shoulders back and down, tuck your bottom under, and feel a fine, silken thread pull you up from the crown of your head.

36. Instead of dessert after dinner, **serve cheese on a plate** and enjoy it spread on bread. You might also have a small bunch of grapes or finely sliced apple, and a bowl of shelled walnuts.

37. Investigate 'main course' **salads which have the wow-factor**. Instead of begrudgingly eating your salad leaves (which I sometimes do), you will look forward to them. Additions such as toasted nuts or seeds, grated or sliced cheese, and a hot component makes all the difference.

38. **Use everything you own**. Save *nothing* for a special occasion, whether dishes or clothing. Enjoy it all. Sure there will be items you use more and some that are used less. But overall, try to use everything you own regularly. If your prettiest vintage wine glasses are covered in a

fine coating of dust at the back of your cupboard, you may as well donate them. And if something is damaged while in use, well at least it lived a full life.

39. Curate **small everyday luxuries** that your European alter ego would enjoy such as gourmet tea, exceptional dark chocolate, beautiful tiny notebooks, and pretty candles. *Surround yourself with special treats.*

40. **Remember your *joie de vivre*.** Life will be difficult or sad at times, but you can always make room for the simple joy of living well. Be extra good to yourself at those times. Sleep a lot, eat well, and wear the softest clothing you own. Cosset yourself and remember that the sun continues to shine every day for you, even if it is covered by clouds sometimes.

41. **Expect to be imperfect.** Drifting away from your plans and dreams does not mean you have failed. You are human. When you see you have strayed from your desired lifestyle goals, simply redirect, just like the map on your phone when you take a wrong turn. There is no need for perfection, just always remember your fun goals and turn towards them over and over. This is how you will get there, and enjoy yourself along the way too.

42. If you must be around people who are not your cup of tea, such as certain family members at holiday get-togethers, be **pleasant but distant**. And always ensure you have dressed in a way that makes you feel confident too.

43. Try some of your new changes out **for one day only**, just to see. Cook from scratch at each meal, dress and do your makeup beautifully, or engage in real life rather than via a screen. You don't have to do this forever more, just do it for today.

44. If you are wanting to lose weight, **buy yourself one or two outfits** in your current size that are inexpensive but still feel 'luxe' and make you feel *amazing*. Curate a small wardrobe this way and see how much it helps you remember your goal when you are tempted to go back to the old familiar foods that used to comfort you. Step into your new life with style.

45. Get rid of anything in your home that has **negative energy**, such as a gift from a friend who hurt you. Why torture yourself?

46. '**Dress for the lifestyle you want**, not the one you have.' Step into your ideal Italian girl by dressing how she would dress. Choose the ballet flats she would wear with her jeans and tee-shirt. Spray the sultry perfume on your wrists.

And practice your cat eye makeup!

47. **Nourish yourself in all ways** – with healthy, delicious food, by dressing in a way that feels good, and by your self-talk too. Read books that make you happy, watch movies that move you. There is nothing selfish in this at all, but I know sometimes it can feel that way. There is nothing to be gained from neglecting yourself. Treat yourself with exquisite kindness and love.

48. **Cut out all junk foods** and see how good you feel. If you are used to eating for taste like I am, it is quite a revelation to see the direct link between what you put in your body and how good (or bad) you feel. Some of us need regular reminders of this. I know I do.

49. **Don't preach to others**, but instead go quietly about your business. Upgrade the quality of your life as you practice both your European-style mindset and being in the world as the upleveled you. Show, don't tell, and influence by your actions not your words.

50. Think about **your beautiful future and how wonderful you can make it**. Fall asleep dreaming about this at night. You can have everything your heart desires. Make it happen, claim your ideal French Chic life, and have fun doing so. You don't need any other reason to

justify yourself other than it's what you are drawn to and what you love. That's all!

Life is what you make of it. Paint it as you wish to live it. Dress with intention, do the things you enjoy, and be that bright spark of bliss who illuminates those around them. I sincerely hope you enjoyed this dainty book and found it motivating in a fun and light-hearted way. I trust you will feel inspired to add a little European flavour to your everyday life even more now!

And if you have a moment I would be beyond grateful if you could leave me a review on Amazon. Even a few words is perfect – you don't have to write a lot. A review is the best compliment you can give to an author. It helps others like yourself find my books, and I'd love to get my message of living well through an inspired mindset to as many ladies as possible!

And if you have anything you'd like to say to me personally, please feel free to write:

fiona@howtobechic.com

Maybe you have a book idea for me, want to let me know what you thought of this book, or have even spotted an error. I hope not, but if you do find a typo please let me know!

Think of me as your friend all the way over in New Zealand, cheering you on and dreaming of the good life, just like you. We enjoy creating our dream life out of thin air. We get to do that! We are a small group, but by gosh are we happy. And those practical people, they can't imagine why we are having so much fun. Just carry on and be you. The world needs more dreamers and doers.

With all my best to you, and I look forward to seeing you in my next book!

Fiona

howtobechic.com
fionaferris.com

About the Author

Fiona Ferris is passionate about the topic of living well, in particular that a simple and beautiful life can be achieved without spending a lot of money.

Her books are published in five languages currently: English, Spanish, Russian, Lithuanian and Vietnamese. She also runs an online home study program for aspiring non-fiction authors.

Fiona lives in the beautiful and sunny wine region of Hawke's Bay, New Zealand, with her husband, Paul, their rescue cat Nina, rescue dogs Daphne and Chloe, and their cousin Micky dog.

To learn more about Fiona, you can connect with her at:
howtobechic.com
fionaferris.com
facebook.com/fionaferrisauthor
twitter.com/fiona_ferris
instagram.com/fionaferrisnz
youtube.com/fionaferris

Fiona's other books are listed on the next page, and you can also find them at:
amazon.com/author/fionaferris

Other books by Fiona Ferris

Thirty Chic Days: *Practical inspiration for a beautiful life*

Thirty More Chic Days: *Creating an inspired mindset for a magical life*

Thirty Chic Days Vol. 3: *Nurturing a happy relationship, staying youthful, being your best self, and having a ton of fun at the same time*

Thirty Slim Days: *Create your slender and healthy life in a fun and enjoyable way*

Financially Chic: *Live a luxurious life on a budget, learn to love managing money, and grow your wealth*

How to be Chic in the Winter: *Living slim, happy and stylish during the cold season*

How to be Chic in the Summer: *Living well, keeping your cool and dressing stylishly when it's warm outside*

A Chic and Simple Christmas: *Celebrate the holiday season with ease and grace*

The Original 30 Chic Days Blog Series: *Be inspired by the online series that started it all*

30 Chic Days at Home: *Self-care tips for when you have to stay at home, or any other time when life is challenging*

30 Chic Days at Home Vol. 2: *Creating a serene spa-like ambience in your home for soothing peace and relaxation*

The Chic Author: *Create your dream career and lifestyle, writing and self-publishing non-fiction books*

The Chic Closet*: Inspired ideas to develop your personal style, fall in love with your wardrobe, and bring back the joy in dressing yourself*

The Peaceful Life*: Slowing down, choosing happiness, nurturing your feminine self, and finding sanctuary in your home*

Loving Your Epic Small Life*: Thriving in your own style, being happy at home, and the art of exquisite self-care*

The Glam Life*: Uplevel everything in a fun way using glamour as your filter to the world*

100 Ways *to Live a Luxurious Life on a Budget*

100 Ways *to Declutter Your Home*

100 Ways *to Live a European Inspired Life*

100 Ways *to Enjoy Self-Care for Gentle Wellbeing and a Healthy Body Image*

100 Ways *to be That Girl*

100 Ways *to Be a Chic Success and Create Your Dream Life*